I0032465

Generis

PUBLISHING

Anatomy Q-Bank: Thorax

Hosam Eldeen Elsadig Gasmalla, PhD

Title: Anatomy Q-Bank: Thorax

ISBN: 979-8-88676-113-9

Author: Hosam Eldeen Elsadig Gasmalla, PhD

Cover image: www.pixabay.com

Publisher: Generis Publishing
Online orders: www.generis-publishing.com
Contact email: info@generis-publishing.com

Editor-in-chief
Hosam Eldeen Elsadig Gasmalla
MBBS, M.Sc. PgDip, MHPE, PhD
Assistant Professor of Human Anatomy
Faculty of Medicine, Al-Neelain University, Sudan

Contributors:

Abuzar Mubarak Omer M.Sc.
Anatomy Department
Al Fashir University

Khalid Elamin Awad PhD
MBBS, MSc., MHPE, PhD
Assistant professor of Anatomy, Faculty of Medicine
University of Khartoum

Omer Tagelsir Abdalla M.Sc.
Anatomy Department
Omdurman Islamic University

Abdelmoneim Alattaya MD, FRCR.
Consultant Radiologist
Antalya Medical Centre

Mohamed Abdelbagi Mohamed
MBBS, MD
Assistant Professor of Radiology
Al Neelain University

Abbas Gareeballa Abdalla PhD
University of Khartoum

Dedication

To my home: mother, father, sister and my brothers

Preface

This is the first edition of a book that is designed to help medical student to study via solving questions, to get the maximum benefit, one shall study from a rich and knowledgeable textbook first; the questions in this book are grouped into four sections

- <u>Section One</u>: MCQs (A-Type): covers the level of recall in the cognitive domain.
- <u>Section Two</u>: Scenario-Based Questions: the questions are primary MCQs based on given scenarios (Cases) to cover the level of comprehension in the cognitive domain.
- <u>Section Three</u>: Extended Matching Questions EMQs (R-Type)to cover the level of the application of knowledge in the cognitive domain.
- <u>Section Four</u>: Medical Imaging: questions about normal X-ray and CT scan images are provided in this section.

I'm looking forward to the useful and productive feedback from my fellow colleagues and the students.

Acknowledgement

I would like to express my gratitude and appreciation to the generations' teacher: Dr. Abbas Gareeballa who has been helping, supporting and advising me since I was a medical student.

Table of Contents

Questions

Section One: MCQs

Thoracic Wall and the Diaphragm

1. **Which one of the following bones is classified as "long bone"?**
   a. Rib.
   b. Clavicle.
   c. Sternum.
   d. Manubrium.
   e. Thoracic vertebra.

2. **The manubrium forms "atypical" synovial joint with the:**
   a. Clavicle.
   b. 1st costal cartilage.
   c. 2nd costal cartilage.
   d. 1st thoracic vertebra.
   e. Body of the Sternum.

3. **Which one of the following synovial joints is "saddle" type?**
   a. Sternocostal joint.
   b. Interchondral joint.
   c. Costovertebral joint.
   d. Costotransverse joint.
   e. Sternoclavicular joint.

4. **Which one of the following muscles is attached to the posterior surface of the manubrium?**
   a. Thyrohyoid.
   b. Sternohyoid.
   c. Teres minor.
   d. Pectoralis major.
   e. Sternocleidomastoid.

5. **Which one of the following joints of the thorax is considered as primary cartilaginous joint?**
    a. Intervertebral joint.
    b. Costochondral joint.
    c. Costovertebral joints.
    d. Costotransverse joint.
    e. Manubriosternal joint.

6. **Which one of the following is located posterior to the lower-left quadrant of the manubrium:**
    a. The oesophagus.
    b. The arch of the aorta.
    c. The superior vena cava.
    d. Left brachiocephalic vein.
    e. Right brachiocephalic vein.

7. **The sternal angle (angle of Louis) is located at the level of the lower border of the following thoracic vertebra:**
    a. 2nd.
    b. 3rd.
    c. 4th.
    d. 5th.
    e. 6th.

8. **Which one of the following costal cartilages forms a synovial joint with the body of the sternum:**
    a. 1st.
    b. 2nd.
    c. 8th.
    d. 9th.
    e. 10th.

9. **Which one of the following muscles is attached along the anterior surface of the body of sternum:**
    a. Sternocostalis.
    b. Internal oblique.
    c. Pectoralis major.
    d. Rectus abdominis.
    e. Transversus abdominis.

10. Which one of the following structures is located posterior to the right-lower quarter of the body of the sternum:
   a. Aortic valve.
   b. Tricuspid valve.
   c. Ascending aorta.
   d. Pulmonary trunk.
   e. Superior vena cava.

11. What is the artery that provides the main supply to the sternum?
   a. Intercostal artery.
   b. Subclavian artery.
   c. Common carotid artery.
   d. Highest thoracic artery.
   e. Internal thoracic artery.

12. Which one of the following ribs articulates only with one vertebra?
   a. 1st rib.
   b. 3rd rib.
   c. 5th rib.
   d. 7th rib.
   e. 9th rib.

13. Which one of the following ribs has no articulation with the transverse process of the corresponding vertebra?
   a. 4th rib.
   b. 6th rib.
   c. 8th rib.
   d. 10th rib.
   e. 12th rib.

14. Which one of the following ribs is classified as "true" rib?
   a. 7th rib.
   b. 8th rib.
   c. 9th rib.
   d. 10th rib.
   e. 11th rib.

15. Regarding rib fractures, which one of the following ribs is the most vulnerable to fractures:
    a. 1st rib.
    b. 2nd rib.
    c. 7th rib.
    d. 11th rib.
    e. 12th rib.

16. Regarding rib fractures, The weakest part of a rib is:
    a. The head.
    b. The tubercle.
    c. Anterior to the angle.
    d. The anterior part of the shaft.
    e. In-between the head and neck.

17. The cervical rib can exert direct pressure on the _____ of the brachial plexus:
    a. Upper trunk.
    b. Lower trunk.
    c. Anterior cord.
    d. Middle cord.
    e. Posterior cord.

18. A groove posterior to scalene tubercle on the superior surface of the first rib lodges the:
    a. Subclavian vein.
    b. Subclavian artery.
    c. Internal jugular vein.
    d. Brachiocephalic trunk.
    e. Right common carotid artery.

19. Which one of the following muscles is attached to the second rib?
    a. Subclavius.
    b. Scalenus medius.
    c. Levator scapulae.
    d. Scalenus anterior.
    e. Scalenus posterior.

20. The xiphoid process starts ossification at the:
    a. Third year.
    b. Second year.
    c. Sixth month after delivery.
    d. 8th month of the intrauterine life.
    e. 5th month of the intrauterine life.

21. Which one of the following is true about subcostalis muscle?
    a. It spans the ribs posteriorly.
    b. It fans out from the sternum.
    c. It is confined to the lower border of rib 12.
    d. It is well developed in upper region of the thorax.
    e. It belongs to middle layer of the intercostal muscles.

22. The neurovascular bundle that runs in the costal groove of a rib is situated:
    a. Deep to the internal intercostal muscle.
    b. Deep to the external intercostal muscle.
    c. Deep to the innermost intercostal muscle.
    d. Between external and internal intercostal muscles.
    e. Between innermost intercostal muscle and the pleura.

23. The posterior intercostal arteries are branches of:
    a. The thoracic aorta.
    b. The subclavian artery.
    c. The inferior thyroid artery.
    d. The internal thoracic artery.
    e. The superior epigastric artery.

24. The 9th anterior intercostal artery is a branch from:
    a. The subcostal artery.
    b. The subclavian artery.
    c. The musculophrenic artery.
    d. The internal thoracic artery.
    e. The superior intercostal artery.

25. The 1st posterior intercostal artery is a branch from:
    a. The subcostal artery.
    b. The costocervical trunk.
    c. The common carotid artery.
    d. The musculophrenic artery.
    e. The internal thoracic artery.

26. The Left superior intercostal vein drains mainly into the:
    a. Azygos vein.
    b. Hemiazygos vein.
    c. Left subclavian vein.
    d. Left brachiocephalic vein.
    e. Accessory hemiazygos vein.

27. The dermatome presents over the nipple is:
    a. T2.
    b. T4.
    c. T6.
    d. T8.
    e. T10.

28. The diaphragm:
    a. Is made of smooth muscle.
    b. Is the chief muscle for expiration.
    c. Raises the intra-thoracic pressure when it is relaxed.
    d. Is innervated by T3, 4 and 5 segments of the spinal cord.
    e. Expands the intra-abdominal cavity when it is contracted.

29. The right dome of the diaphragm ascends to the level of the _____ during expiration:
    a. 5th rib.
    b. 6th rib.
    c. 7th rib.
    d. 8th rib.
    e. 9th rib.

30. The oesophageal hiatus in the diaphragm transmits:
   a. The azygos veins.
   b. The thoracic duct.
   c. The sympathetic trunks.
   d. Branches of the left gastric vessels.
   e. Branches of the right phrenic nerve.

31. The aortic opening in the diaphragm is located at the level of the _____ thoracic vertebra:
   a. 4th.
   b. 6th.
   c. 8th.
   d. 10th.
   e. 12th.

Mediastinum
(Superior, Anterior and Posterior)

32. Which one of the following is found <u>only</u> in the superior mediastinum:
    a. Trachea.
    b. Vagus nerve.
    c. Thoracic duct.
    d. Descending aorta.
    e. Splanchnic nerves.

33. Which one of the following is found <u>both</u> in the superior and posterior mediastina:
    a. Heart.
    b. Trachea.
    c. Oesophagus.
    d. Phrenic nerve.
    e. Pulmonary trunk.

34. Which one of the following is located in the anterior mediastinum:
    a. Thymus.
    b. Oesophagus.
    c. Arch of aorta.
    d. Descending aorta.
    e. Right atrium of the heart.

35. The thymus in the thorax is related anteriorly to the:
    a. Pleura.
    b. Arch of the aorta.
    c. Superior vena cava.
    d. Internal thoracic artery.
    e. Left brachiocephalic vein.

36. The pulmonary trunk carries deoxygenated blood from the _____ of the heart to the lungs:
   a. Left auricle.
   b. Left atrium.
   c. Right atrium.
   d. Left ventricle.
   e. Right ventricle.

37. The pulmonary trunk is first ascends _____ to the ascending aorta:
   a. Deep.
   b. Inferior.
   c. Superior.
   d. Posterior.
   e. Anterior.

38. The pulmonary trunk divides anterior to the _____ into right and left pulmonary arteries:
   a. Arch of the aorta.
   b. Descending aorta.
   c. Left principle bronchus.
   d. Right principle bronchus.
   e. The bifurcation of the trachea.

39. The left brachiocephalic vein is located posterior to the :
   a. Thymus.
   b. Left subclavian artery.
   c. Brachiocephalic artery.
   d. Left internal thoracic artery.
   e. Left common carotid artery.

40. The hemiazygos vein:
   a. Joins the azygos vein at level of T4.
   b. Crosses anterior to the thoracic duct.
   c. Ascends posterior to the thoracic aorta.
   d. Runs to the right side of the vertebral column.
   e. Is the continuation of the right subcostal vein.

41.The azygos vein:
   a. Drains into the accessory hemiazygos vein.
   b. Is the continuation of the left subcostal vein.
   c. Communicates with the vertebral venous plexuses.
   d. Passes close to the left side of the vertebral column.
   e. Runs through the oesophageal opening of the diaphragm.

42.Which one of the following parts drain lymph into the right lymphatic duct :
   a. Uterus.
   b. Left hand.
   c. Right Foot.
   d. Small intestine.
   e. Right cubital fossa.

43.The thoracic duct:
   a. Inclines into the other side at the level of C7.
   b. Runs posterior to the left sympathetic trunk.
   c. Receives all lymphatics below the diaphragm.
   d. Is formed at the left side of the vertebral column.
   e. It ascends into the thorax through the caval opening.

44.The vagus nerve:
   a. Runs downwards anterior to the roots of the lungs.
   b. Passes through the aortic opening of the diaphragm.
   c. Arises from the thoracic segments of the spinal cord.
   d. Gives parasympathetic supply to the thoracic viscera.
   e. Crosses anterior to the brachiocephalic vein in the left side.

45.The left recurrent laryngeal nerve hooks inferiorly around the:
   a. The azygos vein.
   b. The arch of the aorta.
   c. The left subclavian vein.
   d. The left subclavian artery.
   e. The left brachiocephalic vein.

46. The right phrenic nerve:
   a. Arises from T3, 4 and 5.
   b. Runs close to the apex of the heart.
   c. Descends close to the superior vena cava.
   d. Descends posterior to the root of the lung.
   e. Passes through the aortic opening of the diaphragm.

47. The phrenic nerve gives sensory innervation to:
   a. Visceral pericardium.
   b. Parietal costal pleura.
   c. Parietal mediastinal pleura.
   d. Peripheries of the diaphragm.
   e. Visceral diaphragmatic pleura.

48. The greater splanchnic nerve:
   a. Roots are T11 and T12.
   b. Runs in the anterior mediastinum.
   c. Synapse with the cervical superior ganglion.
   d. Conveys visceral afferent fibers from the stomach.
   e. Consists of postganglionic parasympathetic nerve.

49. The lesser splanchnic nerve:
   a. Roots are T5 and T6.
   b. Is a mixed cranial nerve.
   c. Is preganglionic parasympathetic nerve.
   d. Conveys visceral afferent fibers from the appendix.
   e. Passes through the aortic opening of the diaphragm.

50. The oesophagus:
   a. Begins at the level of C3.
   b. Is entirely made of smooth muscles.
   c. Passes posterior to the descending aorta.
   d. Pierces the diaphragm at the level of T12.
   e. Passes through the posterior mediastinum.

51. The oesophagus is constricted at the level of T10 by the effect of:
    a. Left crus.
    b. Right crus.
    c. Arch of the aorta.
    d. Arch of the azygos.
    e. Left principle bronchus

52. The trachea:
    a. Runs posterior to the oesophagus.
    b. Is located to the left side of azygos.
    c. Extends to the anterior mediastinum.
    d. Is at the right side of the arch of the aorta.
    e. Runs posterior to the brachiocephalic trunk.

Lungs and Pleurae

53. The part of pleura that covers the medial aspects of the lungs is named the _____ pleura:
    a. Costal.
    b. Cervical.
    c. Vertebral.
    d. Mediastinal.
    e. Diaphragmatic.

54. The right and left pleurae come in contact anteriorly at the level of the:
    a. 1st rib.
    b. 2nd costal cartilage.
    c. 6th costal cartilage.
    d. 8th rib.
    e. 10th rib.

55. The diaphragmatic pleura is innervated peripherally by the:
    a. Vagus nerve.
    b. Phrenic nerve.
    c. 1st intercostal nerve.
    d. 2nd intercostal nerve.
    e. 8th intercostal nerve.

56. The parietal pleura:
    a. Is insensitive to pain.
    b. Dips into the lung fissures.
    c. Is attached adherently to the lung surfaces.
    d. Joins the visceral pleura at the hilum of the lung.
    e. Forms the costodiaphragmatic recess with the visceral layer.

57. An accidently inhaled object will most likely be located in the:
    a. Left main bronchus.
    b. Right main bronchus.

c. Left lower segmental bronchiole.
d. Right upper segmental bronchiole.
e. Left inferior segmental bronchiole.

58.Which one of the following structures passes posterior to the lung roots:
   a. The vagus nerve.
   b. The phrenic nerve.
   c. The pulmonary ligament.
   d. The pericardiacophrenic vein.
   e. The pericardiacophrenic artery.

59.Which one of the following structures passes superior to the right lung roots:
   a. The azygos vein.
   b. The arch of the aorta.
   c. The pulmonary ligament.
   d. The internal thoracic artery.
   e. The pulmonary autonomic plexus.

60.The lung roots are located at the level of _____ thoracic vertebrae:
   a. 1st to 2nd
   b. 2nd to 3rd.
   c. 5th to 7th.
   d. 9th to 11th.
   e. 11th to 12th.

61.Which one of the following structures runs anterior to the apex of the lung?
   a. The subclavian artery.
   b. Scalenus medius muscle.
   c. The ventral ramus of C1.
   d. The superior intercostal artery.
   e. The stellate sympathetic ganglion.

62.Which one of the following structures leaves an impression on the mediastinal surfaces of both lungs?
   a. The oesophagus.
   b. The arch of azygos.
   c. The arch of the aorta.

d. The inferior vena cava.

e. The superior vena cava.

The Heart

63. The oblique sinus of the pericardium is found:
   a. Superior to the heart.
   b. Posterior to the right atrium.
   c. Anterior to the left ventricle.
   d. Between the aorta and superior vena cava.
   e. Between the right and left pulmonary veins.

64. The base of the heart is formed mainly by the:
   a. Left atrium.
   b. Right atrium.
   c. Right auricle.
   d. Left ventricle.
   e. Right ventricle.

65. The inferolateral part of the left ventricle constitutes the _____ of the heart:
   a. Base.
   b. Apex.
   c. Right border.
   d. Superior border.
   e. Posterior surface.

66. To listen to the sounds of the mitral valve, doctor should place the stethoscope at the:
   a. Point above the middle of the clavicle.
   b. Medial end of the left second intercostal space.
   c. Medial end of the right second intercostal space.
   d. Left fifth intercostal space at the midclavicular line.
   e. Point just to the left of the lower part of the sternum.

67. Which one of the following arteries supplies the apex heart?
   a. SA nodal.
   b. A.V nodal.
   c. Left marginal.

    d. Right marginal.

    e. Circumflex.

68. Which one of the following arteries is the most susceptible to atherosclerotic occlusion?

    a. Circumflex.

    b. Left marginal.

    c. Right marginal.

    d. Anterior interventricular.

    e. Posterior interventricular.

69. The anterior interventricular artery (anterior descending artery) usually supplies the following:

    a. Most of right ventricle.

    b. The SA node in most of people.

    c. The AV node in most of people.

    d. The diaphragmatic surface of the left ventricle.

    e. The anterior part of the inter-ventricular septum.

70. The right coronary artery supplies the inter-ventricular septum via:

    a. Circumflex artery.

    b. Left marginal artery.

    c. Sinoatrial (SA) nodal artery.

    d. Anterior interventricular artery.

    e. Posterior interventricular artery.

71. Infarction of the anterolateral portion of the right ventricle may be due to an obstruction of:

    a. A.V nodal artery.

    b. The anterior descending artery.

    c. Posterior interventricular artery.

    d. Marginal branch of right coronary artery.

    e. Circumflex branch of left coronary artery.

72. Which one of the following veins drains directly into the right atrium?

    a. Great cardiac vein.

    b. Small cardiac vein.

    c. Middle cardiac vein.

    d. Anterior cardiac vein.

    e. Oblique vein of the left atrium.

73.The parasympathetic innervation of the heart is provided by the:
    a. Vagus nerve.
    b. Phrenic nerve.
    c. Lesser splanchnic nerve.
    d. Greater splanchnic nerve.
    e. Right recurrent laryngeal nerve.

74.The sympathetic innervation of the heart:
    a. Decreases heart rate.
    b. Is derived from the vagi.
    c. Dilates the coronary arteries.
    d. Reduces force of contraction.
    e. Constricts the coronary arteries.

Section Two: Scenario-Based Questions

Clinical Case Scenario (1)

Hamid is 22 years old student; he was brought to the emergency department in Omdurman Military Hospital following road traffic accident, he was driving his motorbike when suddenly a car hit him, on examination he was drowsy, his pulse rate was 100 bpm, BP was 110/70 , the doctor noticed that there were some contusions to the left side of his chest and a reverse movement of a chest wall segment at that part during spontaneous breathing, after requesting chest X-ray the doctor made the diagnosis of flail chest complicated by haemo-pneumothorax.

After a while he told the resident doctor that he is facing difficulty in breathing, in reassessment his pulse rate became 90 bpm and the blood pressure dropped into 90/60, the left side was hyper-resonance on percussion, on auscultation the breath sounds on that side were muffled.

Answer the following questions:

75. **In this patient, the negative pressure in the pleural cavity has been disrupted due to the effect of the:**
   a. Neurogenic shock.
   b. Cardiogenic shock.
   c. Tear of the parietal pleura.
   d. Outward pull of the chest wall.
   e. Inward elastic recoil of the lung.

76. **The hyper-resonance in the left side is due to the presence of _____ in the pleural cavity:**
   a. Air.
   b. Pus.
   c. Fluids.
   d. Blood.
   e. Mucous.

77.Breath sounds on the left side were muffled due to the:
   a. Slow pulse rate.
   b. Drop of the blood pressure.
   c. Weakness of heart contractility.
   d. Presence of air in the pleural cavity.
   e. Reverse movement of the chest wall.

Clinical Case Scenario (2)

A resident doctor in the emergency medicine department has been called to examine an old patient in the ward of the cardiology, the patient was severely ill, with marked weight loss, on examination pulse rate was 100 bpm, respiratory rate 22 per minute, neck veins were engorged, heart sounds were diminished and the liver was enlarged (hepatomegaly).

The nurse mentioned to the doctor that the patient has been admitted a few days ago and diagnosed as having Myocardial infarction; she also mentioned that he is under chemotherapy.

The history and the signs were strongly suggestive of "cardiac tamponade".

Answer the following questions:

78. The heart sounds were diminished due to the presence of fluids in between the:
    a. Parietal pleura and pericardium.
    b. Fibrous and parietal pericardium.
    c. Visceral and parietal pericardium.
    d. Pericardium and posterior mediastinum.
    e. Pericardium and sterno-pericardial ligament.

79. The neck veins were engorged due to the congestion in the:
    a. Azygos vein.
    b. Hemiazygos vein.
    c. Superior vena cava.
    d. Left subclavian vein.
    e. Accessory hemiazygos vein.

80. The liver was enlarged due to congestion in the:
    a. Hemiazygos vein.
    b. Inferior vena cava.
    c. Left brachiocephalic vein.
    d. Right brachiocephalic vein.
    e. Right internal thoracic vein.

Clinical Case Scenario (3)

Mustafa is 65 years old teacher brought to the E.R complaining of severe and sharp chest pain, he told the resident doctor that the pain was initially in his shoulder, he was known hypertensive and heavy smoker for 10 years.

ECG showed ST segment elevation in V1, V2 and V3, after work up the doctor made the diagnosis of myocardial infarction.

Answer the following questions:

81. The referred pain in his shoulder is due to the interference of the _____ nerve with the autonomic innervation of the heart:
   a. Vagus.
   b. Phrenic.
   c. Intercostobrachial.
   d. Anterior intercostal.
   e. Recurrent laryngeal.

82. From the mentioned leads on ECG, which artery could be affected?
   a. Circumflex.
   b. Left marginal.
   c. Right marginal.
   d. Anterior interventricular.
   e. Posterior interventricular.

Clinical Case Scenario (4)

Ahmed is 6 years old. He was brought to the Ibraheem Malik hospital; his mother told the resident doctor that he is complaining of repeated chest infections, examination revealed failure to thrive.

Investigations showed congested lung. The diagnosis of Patent Ductus Arteriosus (PDA) was made and plan for surgery was put to action.

After surgery the mother noticed that there is a change in voice of her child.

83. **The failure to thrive due to PDA in this patient can be explained by the effect of the direction of the blood from _____ to _____:**
    a. Pulmonary veins to aorta.
    b. Aorta to pulmonary veins.
    c. Aorta to pulmonary artery.
    d. Pulmonary arteries to aorta.
    e. Pulmonary artery to pulmonary veins.

84. **The repeated chest infections can be explained by lung congestion due to the effect of the gush of blood into the lung from the:**
    a. Aorta.
    b. Right atrium.
    c. Pulmonary vein.
    d. Pulmonary artery.
    e. Superior vena cava.

85. **The change of voice in this patient is due to mistakenly ligated:**
    a. Right vagus nerve.
    b. Left phrenic nerve.
    c. Right phrenic nerve.
    d. Left recurrent laryngeal nerve.
    e. Right recurrent laryngeal nerve.

Section Three: Extended Matching Questions

Movements of the thoracic wall

- **Options:**
    a. Trapezius.
    b. Pectoralis minor.
    c. Scalenus anterior.
    d. Contracted diaphragm.
    e. Relaxed of the diaphragm.
    f. Internal intercostal muscle.
    g. External intercostal muscle.

- **For each movement (or result of movement) described below, select the correct acting muscle from the options (above) that performs the movement (or leads to the result), some of the options may not be used and some of them may be used more than once.**

86. Increase in the intra-abdominal pressure.
87. Elevation of the ribs during deep inspiration.
88. Fixation of the 1st rib during deep inspiration.
89. Increase in the vertical dimension of the thorax.
90. Decrease in the vertical dimension of the thorax.
91. Maintaining the intercostal space during inspiration.
92. Maintaining the intercostal space during expiration.

Blood supply of the heart

- **Options:**
  - a. SA nodal artery.
  - b. Circumflex artery.
  - c. Right marginal artery.
  - d. Anterior interventricular artery.
  - e. Posterior interventricular artery.

- **For each patient with ST-Elevation Myocardial Infarction (STEMI) described below, select the correct coronary artery (above) that when occluded leads to the described conditions of (STEMI), some of the options may not be used and some of them may be used more than once.**

93. Inferior infarction, ST-Elevation at Leads II, III and AVF.
94. Anteroseptal infarction, ST-Elevation at V1 and V3.
95. Posterior infarction, ST-Elevation at V1 and V2.

Figure (1): Chest X-Ray

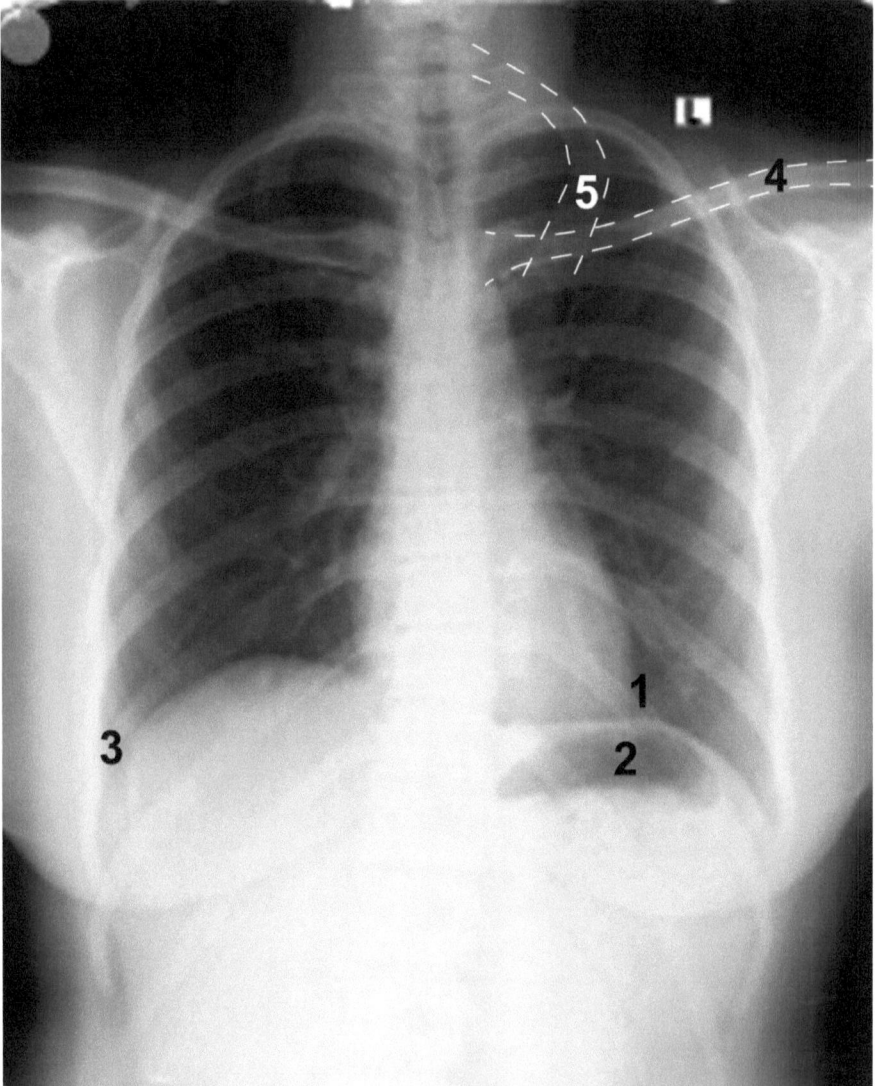

Figure (2): CT scan

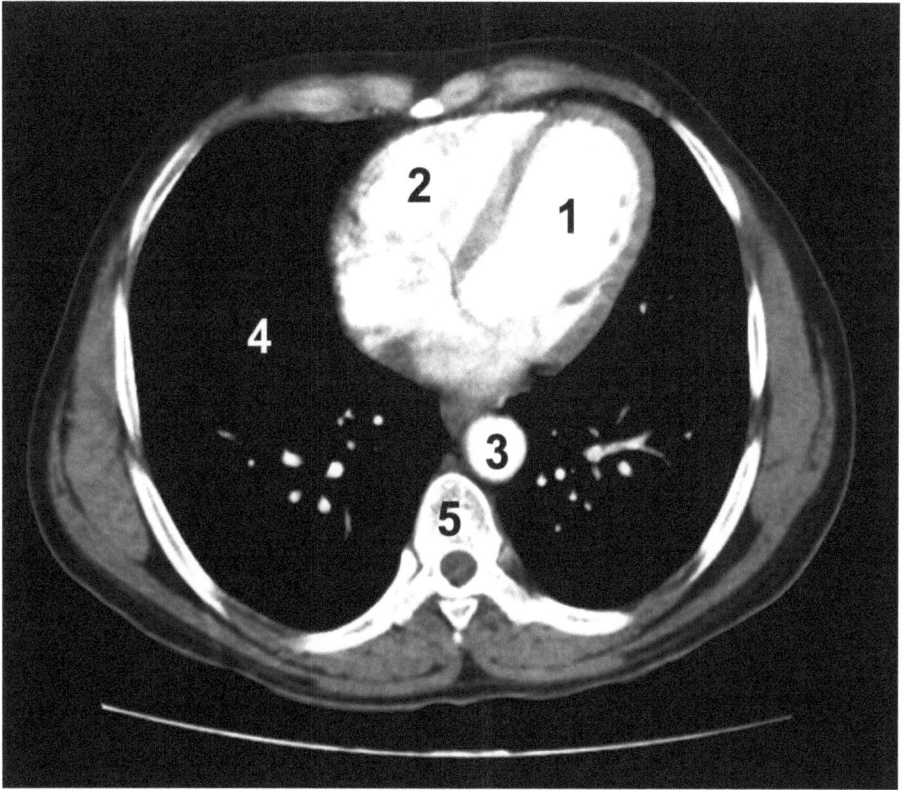

On the previous pages there are two radiological images: Chest X-ray and Axial Chest CT scan, both representing normal appearance of the chest, study them carefully and answer the following questions:

Figure (1): Chest X-Ray

This is a posterior-anterior view of a normal plane chest X-ray, identify the following structures:

96. This part of the heart (1).

97. This space which is filled with air (2).

98. The space (3).

99. Bones (4) and (5).

Figure (2): CT scan

This is a normal CT scan of the thorax: axial section through the heart, identify the following structures:

100. The parts of the heart (1) and (2).
101. The structures (3), (4) and (5).

Answers

Section One: MCQs

Thoracic Wall and the Diaphragm

1. The ribs, manubrium and boy of sternum are flat bones, the vertebrae are irregular and the clavicle is a long bone.

2. **The manubrium is articulated through 7 joints with:**
   - Right and left clavicles: Sternoclavicular joint: synovial joint.
   - Right and left 1st costal cartilages: Sternocostal joints: primary cartilaginous joint.
   - Right and left 2nd costal cartilages: Sternocostal: synovial joint.
   - The sternum: Manubriosternal: secondary cartilaginous joint.
   - No joint exists between the manubrium and any vertebra.

3. **The details about these joints are as follow:**
   - Sternocostal joint: articulation is between the 2nd to 7th costal cartilages with the sternum: Synovial plane joints (the articulation between the 1st costal cartilage and manubrium forms a primary cartilaginous joint).
   - Interchondral joint: articulation is between costal cartilages of 6th and 7th, 7th and 8th, and 8th and 9th: Synovial plane joints.
   - Costovertebral joint: articulation is between the head of the rib and the body of the vertebra: Synovial plane joint.
   - Costotransverse joint: between the tubercle of the rib and the transverse process of the vertebra: Synovial plane joint
   - Sternoclavicular joint: this is "atypical" synovial joint because of the presence of a disc of fibrocartilage that divides the joint cavity into two separate compartments; this joint is classified as "saddle" or "double-plane" joint.

4. **The muscles attachments to the manubrium are as follow:**
   - Sternohyoid and sternothyroid attached are posteriorly (sternohyoid in more superior position).
   - Pectoralis major and sternocleidomastoid are attached anteriorly (sternocleidomastoid in more superior position).

5. **The types of the thoracic joints are as follow:**
   - Costovertebral joints and Costotransverse joint: are synovial.
   - Manubriosternal joint and Intervertebral joint: secondary cartilaginous.
   - Costochondral joint: is primary cartilaginous.

6. **The following structures are related to the posterior surface of the manubrium:**
   - **Posterior to the right side:**
     - Right brachiocephalic vein: upper-right.
     - The superior vena cava: lower right.
   - **Posterior to the left side:**
     - Left brachiocephalic vein: upper left.
     - The arch of the aorta: lower left.
   - The oesophagus doesn't relate to the manubrium, it is separated from it by the tributaries of the superior vena cava, the branches of the arch of the aorta and the trachea (in order form anterior to posterior).

7. **The sternal angle** [angle of Louis: named after Antoine Louis, a French surgeon and physiologist, (1723 - 1792)] is an angle formed at the junction between the manubrium and sternum (manubriosternal joint), it lies at the level of the lower border of T4, it is used as landmark to identify: the 2nd costal cartilage, the bifurcation of the trachea, the pulmonary trunk, the anterior and posterior ends of the arch of the aorta.

8. **Types of joints:**
   - The 1st costal cartilage articulates with the manubrium (not the body of the sternum) to form a primary cartilaginous joint.
   - The 2nd costal cartilage articulates with both the manubrium and the body of sternum forming a synovial joint.
   - The 8th to 10th costal cartilages form synovial joints, but with other costal cartilages: 7th and 8th, 8th and 9th and 9th and 10th (Interchondral joints).

9. **The muscle attachment to the body of sternum (and xiphoid process) is as follow:**
   - **Body of sternum:**
     - **Anterior surface**: Pectoralis major.
     - **Posterior surface**: Transversus thoracis (sternocostalis).
   - **Xiphoid process:**
     - **Anterior surface**: Rectus abdominis and the aponeuroses of external and internal oblique.
     - **Lower border**: The aponeuroses of internal oblique and transversus abdominis are attached to its borders.

10. **The structures that lie behind the body of the sternum:**
    - Upper third: Ascending aorta.
    - The upper part of the
      - Right edge: Superior vena cava
      - Left edge: Pulmonary trunk.
    - The middle of the left edge: Aortic valve.
    - Lower right quadrant: Tricuspid valve.

11. **The main arterial supply to the sternum** is derived from the internal thoracic artery. The artery arises from the first part of subclavian artery, it runs downwards posterior to the clavicle and the 1st costal cartilage, it runs posterior to the upper six costal cartilages just lateral to the sternum, at the level of the 6th costal cartilage it divides into **superior epigastric** and the **musculophrenic** arteries, It supplies the sternum and the upper six intercostal spaces.

12. **The ribs are classified into "typical" and "atypical" ribs according to certain features.**
    - **Features of "typical" rib:**
      - **Head**: two demi-facets to articulate with the bodies of two adjacent vertebrae.
      - **Neck**.
      - **Tubercle**: articulates with the transverse process of the corresponding vertebra.
      - **Angle**.
      - Characteristic features of the **shaft**:
        - Two borders: superior and inferior.

- Two surfaces: inner and outer surfaces.
  - **Costal groove**: at the lower part of the inner surface.
- The first rib is an "atypical" rib; it has:
  - Only **one facet on its head** and doesn't articulate with two vertebrae.
  - **Superior and inferior surfaces** (instead of inner and outer).
  - **Inner and outer borders** (instead of superior and inferior).
  - A **tubercle on its superior surface** for the attachment of the Scalenus anterior muscle.

13. **The ribs articulate with the transverse process of the corresponding vertebrae through their tubercles**. The tubercle has two parts (smooth and rough):
    - The smooth part forms the synovial joint between the rib and transverse process.
    - The rough part gives attachment to the ligament.
    - The eleventh and twelfth ribs are "atypical" ribs, partly because they have **no tubercles**, so they **do not articulate** with the transverse process of the vertebrae.

14. **The ribs are classified into true, false and floating according to their attachment to the sternum**.
    - **The true ribs** are attached to the sternum directly by their costal cartilages. They are from the 1st to the 7th rib.
    - **The false ribs** are attached through their costal cartilages to the costal cartilages of the above ribs, they don't have direct contact with the sternum, they are the 8th, 9th and 10th.
    - **The floating ribs** have no attachment to the sternum (either direct or indirect), they are the 11th and 12th ribs.

15. **The middle ribs are the most vulnerable to fractures,** the first ribs (three or four) are deeply situated and protected by the pectoral muscles and scapula and its muscles, the lower ribs are floating and thus can move with the impact.

16. **The weakest part of a rib** is just anterior to the angle, but direct impact may fracture a rib at any point.

17. **The cervical rib** developmentally is the costal element of the 7th cervical vertebra (it arises from the anterior tubercle of its transverse process), cervical ribs occurs in about 0.5% of people, they are more common than lumbar ribs, the cervical rib can be articulated with the first rib (or its costal cartilage) or connected to it with a fibrous band, it can exert pressure on the lower trunk of the brachial plexus producing sensory and motor symptoms (read about Klumpke's palsy).

18. **The superior surface of the first rib shows two grooves:** the groove that lies anterior to the scalene tubercle lodges the subclavian vein, the groove that lies posterior to the scalene tubercle lodges the subclavian artery, the scalene tubercle serves as attachment for scalenus anterior muscle, which separates the vein and the artery.

19. **Origins, insertions and actions:**
    - **Subclavius**: is attached to the First costal cartilage and the clavicle. It supports the clavicle.
    - **Levator scapulae**: runs from the Transverse processes of first four cervical vertebrae to the Medial border of scapula in which it raises it.
    - **Scalenus anterior, medius and posterior** they all originate from the transverse process of most of the cervical vertebrae (with some variations), and they all insert into the first rib except the scalenus posterior which is inserted into the second rib, their action is to elevate their corresponding ribs.

20. **The xiphoid process** starts ossification at the third year, but remains as cartilage mostly and its ossification is completed around the age of 40.

21. The inner most intercostal muscles are two in number and they form one layer.
    - **Sternocostalis** extends from the lower part of the body of the sternum, xiphoid process and adjacent costal cartilages of the true ribs to be inserted into lower border of the costal cartilages of ribs III to VI.

- **Subcostalis** muscle extends from the internal surfaces of one rib to the internal surface of the second or the third rib below. It is well developed in the lower region of the thorax than the upper region.

22. **The neurovascular bundle** that runs in the costal groove of a rib is situated deep to internal intercostal muscle; that is between innermost and internal intercostal muscle.

23. **The structures in the posterior intercostal spaces** are supplied by the posterior intercostal arteries, branches from the descending abdominal aorta.

24. **The structures in the anterior intercostal spaces** are supplied by the anterior intercostal arteries, they branch out (directly) from the internal thoracic arteries at the upper six intercostal spaces; they branch out from the musculophrenic artery (a branch from the internal thoracic) to supply the lower intercostal spaces, starting from the seventh.

25. **The superior intercostal artery** is a branch of the costocervical trunk (from the subclavian artery), it supplies the 1st and 2nd posterior intercostal spaces.

26. **The left superior intercostal vein** drains the 2nd and 3rd left posterior intercostal veins. It runs across the left side of the arch of the aorta lateral to the left vagus nerve and deep (medial) to the phrenic nerve. It drains into the left brachiocephalic vein.

27. **T2** dermatome overlies the manubrium, **T4** overlies the nipples and **T10** overlies the umbilicus.

28. **Questions 27, 28, 29 and 30: The diaphragm** is a musculotendinous partition between the thorax and abdomen.
    - It is convex towards the thorax and concave towards the abdominal cavity.
    - The right dome of the diaphragm ascends to the level of the 5th rib during expiration.
    - Several structures pass from and to the thorax through the diaphragm.
    - **The caval opening:**

- o**Location**: the central tendon.
  - o**Level**: T8 vertebra.
  - o**Transmits**: The IVC, the right phrenic nerve and few lymphatic vessels.
- **The oesophageal opening:**
  - o**Location** : right crus (muscular part)
  - o**Level**: T10 vertebra.
  - o**Transmits**: The oesophagus, the anterior and posterior vagal trunks and the left gastric vessels.
- **The aortic opening:**
  - o**Location** : posterior to the diaphragm
  - o**Level**: T12 vertebra.
  - o**Transmits**: The aorta, the thoracic duct and the azygos vein.
- **Innervation**:
  - o**Sensory**: the phrenic nerve at the centre and the intercostal nerves at the peripheries.
  - o**Motor**: the phrenic nerve.
- **Function**: It is the chief muscle for inspiration.
- When it contracts, it goes down, leading to
  - oIncrease in the pleural cavity (pleural space).
  - oDecrease in the intra-thoracic pressure.

29. See answer (27) above.

30. See answer (27) above.

31. See answer (27) above.

Mediastinum
(Superior, Anterior and Posterior)

32. **Questions 31, 32 and 33: The mediastinum** is the space between the lungs, it is divided into superior and inferior mediastina by an imaginary line that extends from the angle of Louis anteriorly to a point between T4 and T5, the inferior mediastinum is further divided into anterior, middle and posterior mediastina.

- **Superior mediastinum: structures:**
  - Trachea.
  - Oesophagus.
  - Right and left brachiocephalic veins.
  - Arch of the azygos.
  - Superior vena cava.
  - Arch of the aorta and its three branches.
  - Pulmonary trunk.
  - Vagus, recurrent laryngeal and phrenic nerves.
  - The upper part of the thymus.
- **Posterior mediastinum: structures:**
  - Esophagus.
  - Azygos system of veins.
  - Sympathetic chains.
  - Thoracic splanchnic nerves.
  - Thoracic duct and right lymphatic trunk.
- **Middle mediastinum: structures:**
  - The heart and pericardium.
- **Anterior mediastinum: structures:**
  - Thymus.

33. **See answer (31) above.**

34. **See answer (31) above.**

35. **The thymus** is a primary lymphoid organ, it is responsible of production of T-Lymphocytes; it is located in the superior mediastinum and consists of two lobes joint together by connective tissue, the lower part of the thymus

is extended to the anterior mediastinum down to the level of the 4th costal cartilage. (Note that the question states this: "the thymus in the thorax".. this is because the thymus has an extensions into the neck sometimes, and the question is focusing on the thorax).

- **Relations (in the thorax):**
  - o**Anteriorly**: the manubrium and the internal thoracic vessels.
  - o**Posteriorly**: the left brachiocephalic vein (above),the arch of the aorta (below) and the superior vena cava (to the right).
  - o**Laterally**: pleura.

36. **Questions 35, 36 and 37: the pulmonary trunk** carries deoxygenated blood from the right ventricle of the heart into the lungs, as it does so, it ascends anterior to the ascending aorta, then to the left side of it, it bifurcates into right and left pulmonary arteries inferior to the arch of the aorta and anterior to the left principle bronchus.

37. **See answer (35) above.**

38. **See answer (35) above.**

39. **The left brachiocephalic vein** is longer than the right (owing to the position of the superior vena cava in the right side), it starts posterior to the sternal end of the left clavicle and ends by joining the right brachiocephalic vein to form the superior vena cava at the medial end of the first right costal cartilage, during its course is runs anterior to all the branches of the arch of the aorta and posterior to the sternohyoid and sternothyroid muscles and the thymus.

40. **The hemiazygos vein** is located posteriorly at the left side, it is formed from the lower three posterior intercostal veins, the left ascending lumbar and subcostal veins, it ascends posterior to the thoracic aorta and to the left side of the vertebral column to the level of T9, then it crosses posterior to the aorta and the thoracic duct to join the Azygos vein.

41. **The azygos vein**:
- It is formed by the union of the right ascending lumbar vein and the right subcostal vein.

- It leaves the abdomen to get into the thoracic cavity through the aortic opening in the diaphragm.
- It ascends close to the right side of the vertebral column.
- Receives the hemiazygos and the accessory hemiazygos veins.
- It arches over the root of the right lung to drain into the superior vena cava.
- It communicates with the posterior intercostal veins and the vertebral venous plexuses.
- It receives the mediastinal, oesophageal, and bronchial veins.

42. **The right lymphatic duct** receives the right jugular, subclavian, and Broncho-mediastinal trunks. It drains the right upper limb and the right side of the thorax, head and neck. Into the right brachiocephalic vein.

43. **The thoracic duct:**
    - It is the largest lymphatic duct in the body.
    - It is formed at the right side of T12 or L1 as confluence of lymph trunks which is saccular in shape (called: the cisterna chyli).
    - It ascends into the thorax through the aortic opening with the aorta on its left side and the azygos vein on its right side.
    - It ascends in the posterior mediastinum and inclines to the left at the level of T4/T5.
    - Then it arches more to the left at the level of the transverse process of C7.
    - The arch of the thoracic duct crosses anterior to the vertebral artery, left sympathetic trunk, thyrocervical trunk and the left phrenic nerve.
    - Then it runs down anterior to the left subclavian artery to join the junction of the (the left subclavian and internal jugular) veins.
    - It drains lymph from all the body except the right upper limb and the right side of the thorax, head and neck.

44. **The vagus nerve:**
    - It is the 10th cranial nerve.
    - Gives rise to parasympathetic innervation to the thoracic and most of the abdominal viscera.
    - **The right vagus:**
        o Crosses anterior to the first part of subclavian artery.

- As it descends it moves gradually from the right side of the right brachiocephalic vein to its posteromedial side.
- It runs in close relation to the right lung (and pleura) but lower down it gets separated from it by the azygos vein.
- **The left vagus:**
  - Enters the thorax between the left common carotid and subclavian arteries.
  - Crosses posterior to the left brachiocephalic vein.
  - Runs across the left side of the arch of the aorta, in which it gets crossed of the left side by the left superior intercostal vein, the phrenic never here is located anterior to the vagus.
- **Right and left vagi:**
  - Run downwards posterior to the roots of the lungs.
  - Enter the abdomen through the oesophageal opening of the diaphragm.

45. **The left recurrent laryngeal nerve** curves below the arch of the aorta, the right recurrent laryngeal nerve curves below the right subclavian artery, both are branches form the vagi; they turn around and ascend between the trachea and oesophagus (tracheoesophageal groove) to reach the larynx in the neck and supply it with motor and sensory fibers.

46. **Questions 45 and 46: The phrenic nerves** roots are C3, 4 and 5; they enter the thoracic cavity by passing between the subclavian artery the brachiocephalic vein in each side, each one of them runs down wards anterior to the roots of the lungs, they are the sole motor supply to the diaphragm, they also give rise to sensory fibers to the center of the diaphragm and the parietal mediastinal pleura.
- **The left phrenic nerve:**
  - Runs across the arch of the aorta.
  - Passes along the left side of the arch of the aorta anterior to the left vagus nerve.
  - Crosses on the right side to the left superior intercostal vein.
  - Runs downwards close to the left atrium and ventricle.
  - It pierces the diaphragm just to the left of the pericardium.
- **The right phrenic nerve:**
  - Passes along the right side of the superior vena cava and the right atrium.

o Passes to the abdomen through caval opening of the diaphragm.

47. See answer (45) above

48. Questions 47 and 48:
- **The splanchnic nerves are three**: greater, lesser and least.
  - o **They consist** of sympathetic preganglionic efferent and visceral afferent fibres.
  - o **They run** in the posterior mediastinum.
- **The greater splanchnic nerve:**
  - o **Roots are**: T5, 6, 7, 8 and 9.
  - o **Ends**: most of the sympathetic preganglionic efferent end by synapse at the coeliac ganglion. The rest of the preganglionic fibers synapse at the aorticorenal ganglion and suprarenal medulla.
  - o **Conveys** visceral afferent fibers from the gallbladder and stomach.
- **The lesser splanchnic nerve:**
  - o **Roots are**: T10 and 11.
  - o **Ends**: most of the sympathetic preganglionic efferent end by synapse at the aorticorenal ganglion.
  - o **Conveys** visceral afferent fibers from the appendix.
- **The least splanchnic nerve:**
  - o **Root is**: T12.
  - o **Ends**: most of the sympathetic preganglionic efferent end by synapse at the renal plexus.

49. See answer (47) above.

50. The oesophagus is a muscular tube starts as a continuation of the pharynx at the level of C6 (the level of the cricoid cartilage), its upper part is made of skeletal muscles, the lower part is made of smooth muscles and it is mixed in between, it runs downwards posterior to the trachea; in the posterior mediastinum it starts shifting gradually to become anterior to the descending thoracic aorta, it leaves the thorax by passing through its own opening in the diaphragm at the level of T10, it ends by entering the stomach at the level of T11.

51.The constrictions of the oesophagus are three:

- Where it is crossed by the arch of the aorta.
- Where it is crossed by the left principal bronchus.
- As it passes through the diaphragm, the constriction is due to its left inclination against the traction of the right crus of the diaphragm.

52.The trachea runs anterior to the oesophagus in the superior mediastinum, on its right side runs the brachiocephalic trunk and the azygos arches to enter the superior vena cava, the arch of the aorta is on its left side.

Lungs and pleurae

53. The pleura is named according to its location:
- **Cervical:** covers the dome (apex) of the lung.
- **Mediastinal:** covers the mediastinal (medial) surface of the lung.
- **Costovertebral:** lines the thoracic wall and the thoracic vertebrae internally.
- **Diaphragmatic:** covers the diaphragmatic (inferior) surface of the lung.

54. Surface anatomy of the pleurae:
- **Anterior view:**
  - o **Sternoclavicular joints:** both plural edges pass downwards from behind the joint.
  - o **2nd costal cartilage:** they meet in the midline at this level.
  - o The pleural edges pass **vertically downwards** to:
    1. The **6th costal cartilage** (right pleura).
    2. The **4th costal cartilage** (left pleura).
  - o The pleural edges cross the **8th rib** in the **mid-clavicular line.**
- **Lateral view:**
  - o The pleural edges cross:
    1. The **10th rib** in the **mid-axillary line.**
    2. The **12th rib** posterolaterally.

55. Innervation of the pleura:
- **Costal pleura**: corresponding intercostal nerves.
- **Mediastinal pleura**: phrenic nerves.
- **Diaphragmatic pleura**: corresponding intercostal nerves peripherally and phrenic nerves centrally.

56. The parietal pleura (unlike the visceral pleura) is sensitive to pain, it lines the thoracic wall internally and the diaphragm superiorly, a space between it and visceral pleura is named the (pleural cavity), the costal and diaphragmatic layers of the parietal pleura form the costodiaphragmatic recess, it joins the visceral pleura at the hilum of the lung.

57.An accidently inhaled object will most likely enter the right principal bronchus: it is wider, shorter and more vertical than the left one.

58.Questions 57, 58 and 59: The lung roots:
- This term is referred to the following structures going in and out of the lung at its hilum, collectively:
    o The principal bronchus.
    o The pulmonary artery.
    o The pulmonary veins (two).
    o The bronchial vessels.
    o The pulmonary autonomic plexus.
    o Lymphatics.
- The lung roots are located at the level of the 5th to 7th thoracic vertebrae.
- **Anterior relations:**
    o The phrenic nerve.
    o The pericardiacophrenic vessels.
    o The anterior pulmonary plexus.
- **Posterior relations:**
    o The vagus nerve.
    o The posterior pulmonary plexus.
- **Superiorly:**
    o **Left lung roots:** The arch of the aorta.
    o **Right lung roots:** The arch of the azygos.
- **Inferiorly**: the pulmonary ligament.

59.See answer (57) above.

60.See answer (57) above.

61.Anatomical relations of the apex of the lung:
- **Anteriorly**: The subclavian artery and scalenus anterior muscle anterior to the artery.
- **Posteriorly**:
    o The stellate sympathetic ganglion.
    o The ventral ramus of C1.
    o The superior intercostal artery.
- **Laterally**: Scalenus medius muscle.

62. Impressions on the lung:

- **Impressions on the right lung are for:**
  - Superior vena cava.
  - Arch of azygos.
  - Oesophagus.
  - First rib.
  - The heart.
- **Impressions on the left lung are for:**
  - Arch of the aorta.
  - Oesophagus.
  - First rib.
  - The heart.

The Heart

63. **The oblique pericardial sinus**: is a wide pocket-like recess in the pericardial cavity posterior to the base (posterior aspect) of the heart.

64. **Questions 64 and 65: The borders and surfaces of the heart** are as follows:
    - **Anterior (sternocostal) surface.**
      - Formed mainly by the right ventricle.
    - **Diaphragmatic (inferior) surface.**
      - Formed mainly by the left ventricle.
    - **Right border**:
      - Formed by the right atrium and extending between the SVC and the IVC.
    - **Inferior border**:
      - Formed mainly by the right ventricle and slightly by the left ventricle.
    - **Left border:**
      - Formed mainly by the left ventricle and slightly by the left auricle.
    - **Superior border**:
      - Formed by the right and left atria and auricles in an anterior view.
    - **The apex of the heart:**
      - Formed by the inferolateral part of the left ventricle.
    - **The base of the heart:**
      - It is the heart's posterior aspect (opposite the apex).
      - Formed mainly by the left atrium.

65. **See answer (64) above.**

66. **Auscultation for heart sounds:**
    - **The tricuspid valve**: just to the left of the lower part of the sternum near the 5th intercostal space.
    - **The mitral valve:** over the apex of the heart in the left 5th intercostal space at the midclavicular line.

- **The pulmonary valve:** over the medial end of the left 2nd intercostal space.
- **The aortic valve:** over the medial end of the right 2nd intercostal space.

67. **Questions 66, 67, 68, 69 and 70: The blood supply of the heart** is derived from two arteries which arise from the ascending aorta: the right and left coronary arteries.
    - **The left coronary** has the following branches:
        - The anterior interventricular artery (The alternative name for this artery is the anterior descending artery LAD) supplies the anterior two thirds of the interventricular septum, most of the ventricles (left and right), conducting system and left ventricle.
        - Left circumflex which runs posteriorly around the left border and supply the posterior surface, before passing posteriorly it gives the Left marginal artery to the apex.
        - SA nodal artery.
    - **Right coronary artery** supplies the right and posterior heart by the following branches:
        - Anterior ventricular arteries for the right atrium and ventricle.
        - The right marginal supplies the right and inferior borders of the heart.
        - Posterior interventricular artery supplies the posterior surface and the AV node by the AV nodal artery.

68. See answer (66) above.

69. See answer (66) above.

70. See answer (66) above.

71. See answer (66) above.

72. Most veins of the heart drain into the **coronary sinus** which in turn drains into the right atrium. these veins are:
    - **The great cardiac vein:** it drains the anterior and left surfaces of the heart.

- **The middle cardiac vein:** joins the great at the posterior surface and drain the posterior aspect of the heart.
- **The small cardiac vein:** comes from the right margin and join the previously mentioned veins forming the coronary sinus.
- **The anterior cardiac vein:** at the anterior surface of the heart, ascends upward on the anterior wall of the right ventricle and atrium then pierces the wall of right atrium to drain directly into it without joining coronary sinus.
- The smallest cardiac veins (**Venae cordis minimae**) are small veins collect the blood and penetrate the wall of the heart to drain into its all champers even the ventricles; here some kind of oxygen shunt occurs because venous blood get mixed with blood of the left ventricle. They are valve-less; they may carry blood in the opposite direction and supply the myocardium.

73. **Questions 72 and 73: The heart is innervated from** the deep and superficial cardiac plexuses; they are located in the mediastinum behind the heart and close to the left bronchus, pulmonary trunk and arch of aorta.
- The cardiac plexuses composed of two sources mainly:
  o **Sympathetic**: from the cervical and upper thoracic sympathetic ganglia (the sympathetic flow to the heart); it accelerates the heart rate, increases the force of contraction and dilates the coronary arteries to enhance the blood flow.
  o **Parasympathetic**: from the vagus nerve, it slows the heart rate to the normal, decreases force of contraction and constricts the coronary arteries.

74. **See answer (72) above.**

Section Two: Scenario-Based Questions

Clinical Case Scenario (1)

75. The pleural cavity which lies between parietal and visceral pleura, must be closed space with a low presser (about 756 mmHg, lower than the atmospheric pressure: 760 mmHg), this negative pressure allows entrance of air into the lung passively without suction effort.
    - Air and blood accumulate within the cavity as a result of trauma to the ribs which leads to tear of pleura, followed by entrance of air and raising of the pressure in the pleural cavity to the level of the atmospheric pressure or above.
        - Difficulty of breathing is due to haemopneumothorax which raises the pressure of pleural cavity and its negativity gets lost and the air won't enter the lung passively; now the patient needs effort to suck the air.
        - Drop of blood pressure is due to bleeding.
    - Pneumothorax :**AIR** within the pleural cavity
    - Haemothorax: **BLOOD** within the pleural cavity.
    - Hydrothorax: **FLUIDS** within the pleural cavity.

76. The pleural cavity must be empty except of trace amount of fluids for lubrication, prevention of friction and normal adhesion of pleurae to prevent lung collapse.
    - **Percussion**: tapping the thorax over the chest wall with the fingers while listening for differences in sound wave conduction to detect the type of sounds in the lungs and neighbouring structures and tissues.
        - o Air filled (**resonant sound**).
        - o Fluid filled (**dull sound**).
        - o **Hyper resonance** due to presence of a lot of air more than the normal amount of the lungs air.

77. Air in the pleural cavity hinders listening to breath sound by auscultation.

Clinical Case Scenario (2)

78. The heart rests over the diaphragm and is covered by tough membrane called the pericardium , the pericardium is composed of two parts:

   o **Fibrous pericardium** is very tough membrane enclosing the heart completely, attaching to the great vessels of the heart and diaphragm to keep the heart in position.

   o **Serous pericardium** is very thin membrane covered the heart deep to the fibrous pericardium and also lines fibrous pericardium from inside, the layer which is directly covered the heart called the **visceral pericardium** and the layer which lines the fibrous pericardium from inside is the **parietal pericardium**.

- Between the visceral and parietal pericardium there is the pericardial cavity, normally containing thin film of fluids for lubrication.
- Abnormal accumulation of fluid within the pericardial cavity leads to cardiac tamponade.
   o **Pericardial effusion**: small amount of fluid in the pericardial cavity.
   o **Cardiac tamponade** (heart compression) : excess and accumulation of large amount fluid which in turn affects the function of the heart (restricts the heart movements) or may cause cardiac arrest.

79. As the fibrous pericardium attaches to the great vessel which are entering and leaving the heart, this attachment cause congestion and narrowing the vessels when the pericardial cavity filled with fluid and blood and also produce heavy pressure over the heart because of the fibrous pericardium is tough and doesn't stretch.

- Due to congestion of the superior vena cava the venous return is affected and decreased, the veins of the neck are engorged with blood.

80. Due to the congestion of the inferior vena cava the venous return from the liver is affected and decreased and the blood accumulated in the liver , this increases the size of liver (hepatomegaly).

Clinical Case Scenario (3)

81. When cardiac cells die during myocardial infarction, pain fibers (visceral) are stimulated.

- These sensory fibers (visceral) follow the course of sympathetic fibers that innervate the heart and enter the spinal cord between TI and TIV levels.
- At this level, afferent nerves (somatic) from spinal nerves T1 to T4 also enter the spinal cord via the posterior roots.
- Both types of afferents (visceral and somatic) ascend to the somatosensory areas of the brain that represent the T1 to T4 levels.
- The brain is unable to distinguish clearly between the visceral sensory distribution and the somatic sensory distribution and therefore the pain is interpreted as arising from the somatic regions rather than the visceral organ.

82. Please read this table:

Artery	ECG leads
Anterior interventricular artery	Chest leads V1 to V4
Right coronary	Limb leads 2, 3 and AVF
Circumflex	Limb leads 1 Chest leads V5 and V6

Clinical Case Scenario (4)

83. Questions 83, 84 and 85:
- **Ligamentum arteriosum** is an embryologic remnant. During embryonic life it was a duct known as ductus arteriosus (duct that connects the arch of the aorta to the left pulmonary artery to bypass the lung), normally it gets closed at birth.
- **Patent ductus arteriosus** is one of the congenital heart diseases. It is a cyanotic heart disease. After birth the pressure in the aorta is higher than that in the pulmonary trunk, so the oxygenated blood from the aorta passes to the pulmonary artery through the patent ductus arteriosus. This has two effects, the first is that the blood passes through the aorta to systemic circulation becomes less than normal and this leads to growth abnormality (failure to thrive), the second is that the blood that passes from the aorta to pulmonary artery leads to lung congestion and repeated chest infections, later on it causes pulmonary hypertension and reverse of the direction of blood.
- In order to correct this condition the ductus arteriosus should be closed, the left recurrent laryngeal nerve should be preserved; otherwise if it is mistakenly ligated change of voice will occur, for this nerve supplies the larynx (voice production organ).

84. See answer (83) above.

85. See answer (83) above.

Section Three: Extended Matching Questions

Movements of the thoracic wall

86. Questions 86, 87, 88, 89, 90, 91 and 92:
    - **The following muscles are active during inspiration**:
        - Contracted diaphragm: it increases the anterio-posterior, transverse and vertical dimensions of the thorax and raises the intra-abdominal pressure.
        - External intercostal muscles: they maintain the intercostal space during inspiration.
    - **The following muscles are active during deep inspiration**:
    - The accessory muscle of respiration: pectoralis major, pectoralis minor and the serratus anterior muscle: they elevate the ribs during deep inspiration.
    - Other accessory muscle of respiration: the scalene muscles: they fix the 1st and 2nd ribs during deep inspiration.
    - The following muscles are active during expiration:
    - The Internal intercostal muscles: maintain the intercostal space during expiration.
    - The diaphragm decreases the dimensions of the thorax upon relaxation.

87. See answer (86) above.

88. See answer (86) above.

89. See answer (86) above.

90. See answer (86) above.

91. See answer (86) above.

92. See answer (86) above.

Blood Supply of the Heart

93. Correlation between the site of infarction and the possibly occluded artery:
ST-Elevation Myocardial Infarction (STEMI)

Site Of infarction	Possibly occluded artery
Inferior infarction, ST-Elevation at Leads II, III and AVF.	Posterior interventricular artery
Anteroseptal infarction, ST-Elevation at V1 – V4.	Anterior interventricular artery
Posterior infarction, ST-Elevation at V1 and V2.	Circumflex artery

94. See answer (93) above.

95. See answer (93) above.

Section Four: Medical Imaging

Figure (1): Chest X-Ray

This is a posterior-anterior (PA) view of a normal chest X-ray, identify the following structures:

96. This part of the heart (1): the Apex

97. This space which is filled with air (2): the fundus of the stomach, the normal stomach bubble should not be confused with free intra-abdominal gas.

98. The space in (3): right costodiaphragmatic recess.

99. Bones in:
- **(4):** left clavicle.
- **(5):** left first rib.

Figure (2): CT scan

This is a normal CT scan of the thorax: axial section through the heart, identify the following structures:

100. The parts of the heart in:
- **(1):** left ventricle.
- **(2):** right ventricle.

101. The structures in:
- **(3):** descending aorta.
- **(4):** right lung.
- **(5):** vertebral body.

References:

1) Drake, Richard L. et al. 2007. *GRAYS anatomy for students*. Elsevier Inc.
2) Ellis, H. 2006. *Clinical Anatomy, Applied anatomy for students and junior doctors*. 11th Ed, Blackwell Publishing Ltd.
3) McMinn, R.M.H. 1997. *LAST'S anatomy regional and applied*. 9th Ed. Churchill Livingstone.
4) Moore, Keith L. and Dalley, Arthur F. 2006. *Clinically Oriented Anatomy*. 5th Ed. Lippincott Williams & Wilkins.
5) Snell, Richard S. 2007. *Clinical Anatomy by Regions*. 8th Ed. Lippincott Williams & Wilkins.
6) Standring S. 2008. *Gray's Anatomy: The Anatomical basis For Clinical Practice*. 39th Ed. Elsevier.

www.ingramcontent.com/pod-product-compliance
Lightning Source LLC
Chambersburg PA
CBHW041312210326
41599CB00003B/85